Sugar Detox Diet

Lose Sugar to Lose Weight

Table of Contents

Introduction

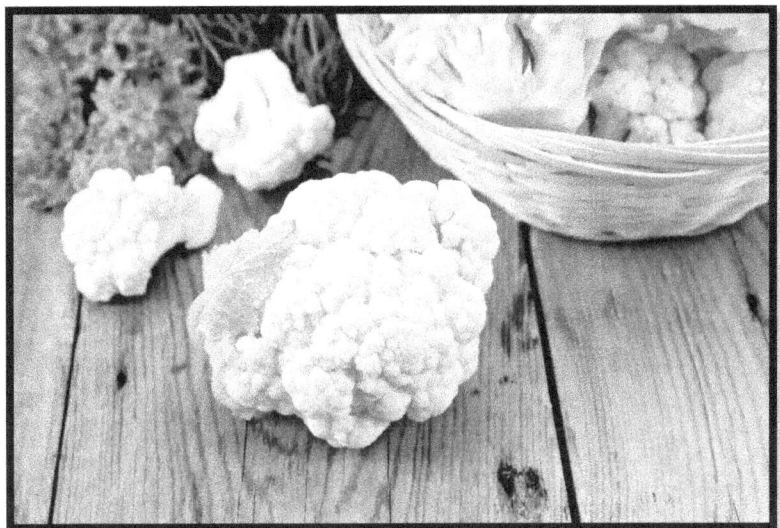

Do you struggle with sugar cravings? Are you having trouble losing weight? You may not realize it, but the answers to these two questions could be related. Countless individuals are addicted to sugar without even realizing it, and it has significant effects on their health. If you consume sugary foods on a regular basis, including foods made with zero-calorie sweeteners, your body has likely formed an addiction to sugar and you could be suffering the effects. In this book, you will learn the basics about what a sugar detox diet is and how it can help you to break your sugar habits and start losing weight. In addition to this information, you will also find a collection of 25 delicious recipes to help you get started on your sugar detox diet.

What is the Sugar Detox Diet?

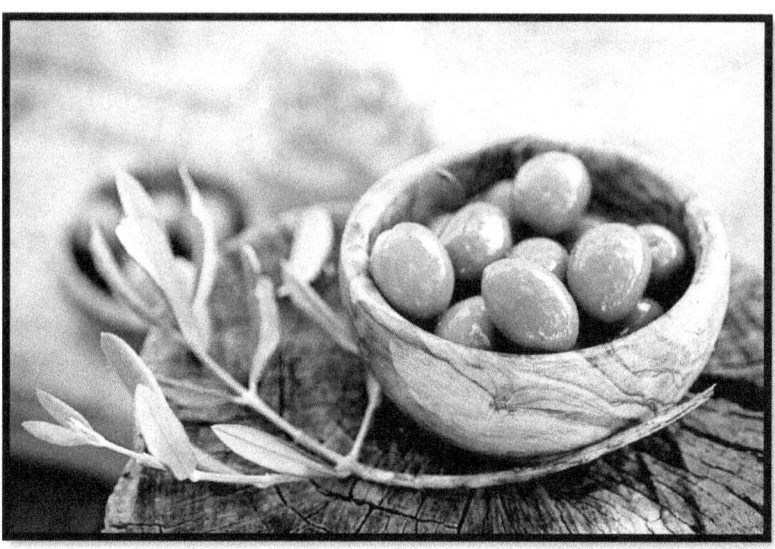

The sugar detox diet is simply a sugar-free diet designed to help cleanse your body of the negative effects of your sugar addiction. Even if you only eat sugar a few times a week, it could be enough to cause an addiction. You may not even realize that there is sugar in some of the foods you eat – it is hidden in canned foods, sauces, frozen dinners, sports drinks, and more. It is estimated that the average American consumers more than 150 pounds of sugar each year. Adding a packet of sugar to your morning coffee or enjoying a sweet dessert once in a while may seem harmless, but even small amounts of sugar add up over time.

The basis of the sugar detox diet is, of course, to get rid of sugar – this means all types of sugar! Not only will you be getting rid of refined sugar like granulated sugar, brown sugar, and powdered sugar but also natural sweeteners like maple syrup and honey. You will also have to give up artificial sweeteners and naturally sweet foods like fruit. The only exceptions to this rule are green apples and under-ripe bananas because these fruits have such a mild sweetness that it is unlikely to trigger cravings and hamper your progress on the sugar detox diet. In addition to avoiding sugar and sweeteners, it is also recommended that you consume only gluten-free grains and full-fat dairy products on the sugar detox diet. This means you will need to avoid low-fat, reduced-fat and fat-free products.

Here is a basic list of the types of foods you will be eating on a sugar detox diet:

- Red meat (all cuts)
- Poultry (all types)
- Eggs
- Fish and seafood
- Leafy greens
- Non-starchy vegetables
- Gluten-free grains
- Beans, chickpeas and lentils
- Whole milk and cream
- Greek yogurt
- Full-fat cheeses
- Nuts and seeds
- Olive and coconut oil
- Almond and coconut flour
- Herbs and spices

*Note: While green apples and under-ripe bananas are allowed on the sugar detox diet, you should enjoy these foods in moderation – no more than one serving per day. You should also limit your intake of starchy vegetables like butternut squash and acorn squash. Avoid refined sugars and flours as well as sweet potato/yams, gluten-containing grains, processed foods, fast food and store-bought condiments.

At this point you may be worried that the sugar detox diet seems pretty extreme. You do have to give up sugar (and all foods containing sugar), but you will find that you still have plenty of options – simply refer to the collection of recipes found in the second half of this book! Additionally, <u>you will experience a variety of healthy benefits, including but not limited to, the following</u>:

- Improved (healthy) weight loss results
- Relief from sugar and carb cravings
- Improved energy levels, relief from chronic fatigue
- Increased stamina and overall wellbeing
- Improved mental clarity and focus
- Better quality of sleep, fewer sleep problems
- Improved skin and hair health

If you are ready to experience these benefits and more for yourself, get started on the sugar detox diet today! The recipes in the following section will help you kick-start your sugar detox diet.

Sugar Detox Diet Recipes

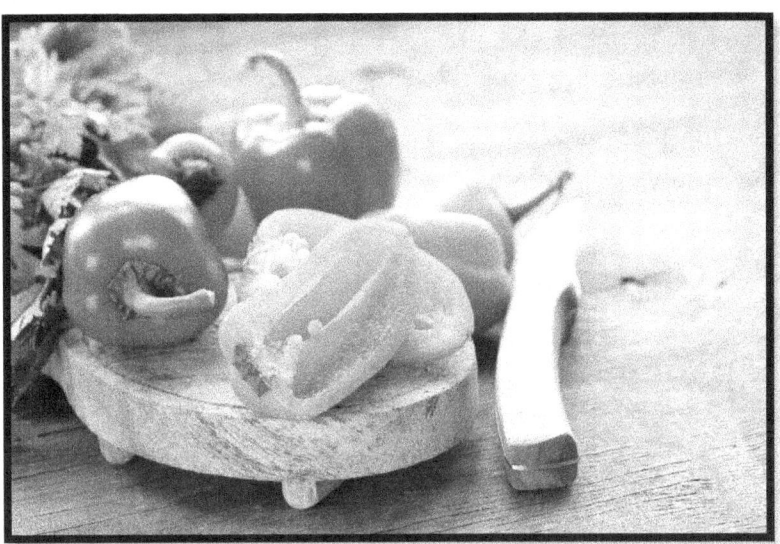

Recipes Included in this Book:

Green Apple Cucumber Smoothie

Servings: 1 to 2

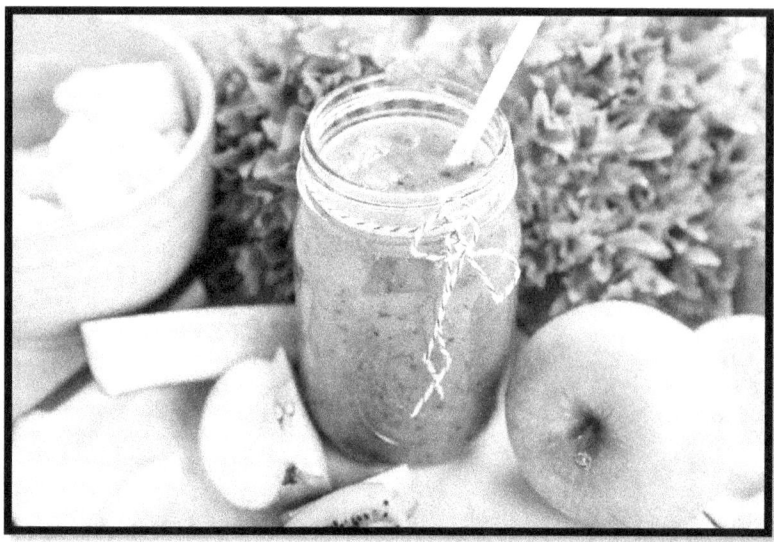

Ingredients:

- 2 medium green apples, cored and chopped
- 1 small seedless cucumber, peeled and diced
- 1 cup water
- ½ cup ice cubes
- 1 tablespoon fresh lemon juice

Instructions:

1. Combine all of the ingredients in a blender.
2. Blend on high speed for 40 to 60 seconds until smooth.
3. Pour into a glass and serve immediately.

Banana Walnut Muffins

Servings: 12

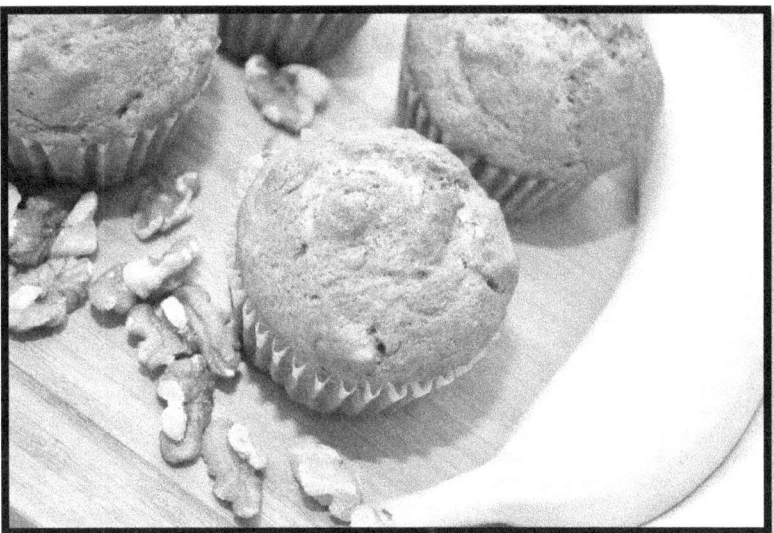

Ingredients:

- 4 medium green bananas, peeled and chopped
- 4 large eggs, whisked
- ½ cup almond butter
- 3 tablespoons unsalted butter, melted
- ½ cup coconut flour
- 1 tablespoon ground cinnamon
- 1 ¼ teaspoon baking powder
- ¾ teaspoon baking soda
- Pinch salt
- ½ cup chopped walnuts

Instructions:

1. Preheat the oven to 350°F and line a muffin pan with paper liners.
2. Combine the bananas, eggs, almond butter, butter and vanilla extract in a food processor.
3. Blend the mixture until smooth.
4. In a mixing bowl, stir together the coconut flour, cinnamon, baking powder, baking soda, and salt.

5. Add the dry ingredients to the wet ingredients in the food processor in small batches, blending smooth between each addition.
6. Transfer the batter to a bowl then fold in the walnuts.
7. Spoon the batter into the prepared pan, filling the cups about 2/3 full.
8. Bake for 20 to 25 minutes until a knife inserted in the center comes out clean.
9. Cool the muffins in the pan for 5 minutes then turn out onto a wire rack to cool completely.

Refreshing Green Smoothie

Servings: 1 to 2

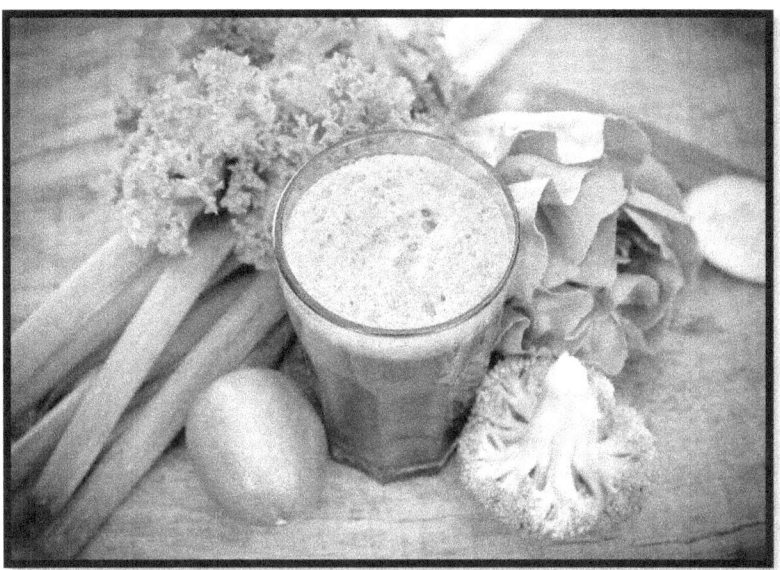

Ingredients:

- 1 small seedless cucumber, peeled and diced
- 1 leave Romaine lettuce, chopped
- 1 leaf curly kale, chopped
- 1 cup chopped broccoli florets
- 1 cup water
- ½ cup ice cubes
- 1 tablespoon fresh lime juice

Instructions:

1. Combine all of the ingredients in a blender.
2. Blend on high speed for 40 to 60 seconds until smooth.
3. Pour into a glass and serve immediately.

Cinnamon Banana Pancakes

Servings: 3 to 4

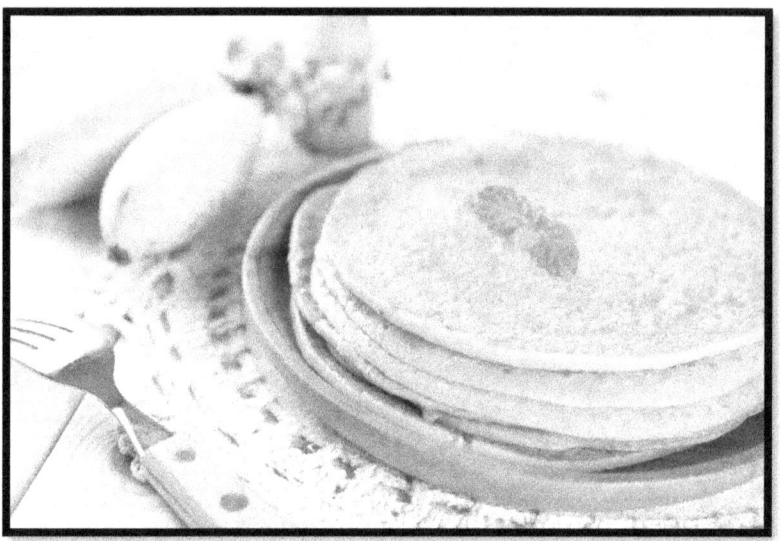

Ingredients:

- ½ cup mashed banana
- 1 cup canned coconut milk
- 3 large eggs, whisked
- ½ teaspoon almond extract
- 1 ¼ cups almond flour
- 3 heaping tablespoons coconut flour
- 1 teaspoon ground cinnamon
- ¾ teaspoon baking soda
- ¼ teaspoon salt

Instructions:

1. Grease and preheat a large skillet over medium-high heat.
2. In a mixing bowl, combine the banana, coconut milk, eggs and almond extract.
3. Whisk until smooth and well combined.
4. In a separate bowl, whisk together the almond flour, coconut flour, baking soda, salt and cinnamon.
5. Add the dry ingredients to the wet and whisk smooth.
6. Spoon the batter into the hot skillet using 2 to 3 tablespoons per pancake.

7. Cook the pancakes for 1 to 2 minutes until browned on the underside then flip and cook for 1 to 2 minute more.
8. Transfer the pancakes to a plate to keep warm and repeat with the remaining batter.

Corned Beef Hash

Servings: 4

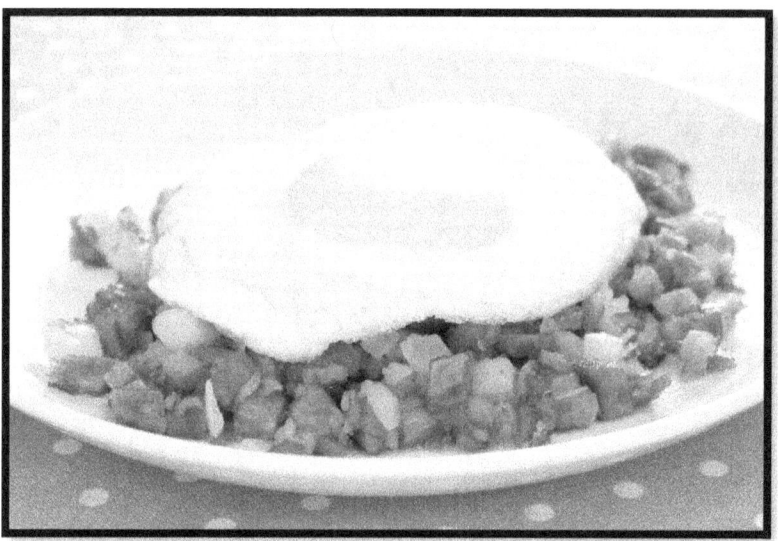

Ingredients:

- 2 tablespoons coconut oil
- 4 cups cooked corned beef, diced
- 1 large yellow onion, chopped
- 1 teaspoon minced garlic
- Pinch dried thyme
- ¼ teaspoon ground cinnamon
- ¼ cup beef broth
- Salt and pepper to taste
- 4 large eggs

Instructions:

1. Heat the oil in a heavy skillet over medium heat.
2. Add the onion and garlic and cook for 6 to 8 minutes until the onion is translucent.
3. Stir in the corned beef, thyme and cinnamon then cook for 1 minute.
4. Add the beef broth then season with salt and pepper to taste.
5. Simmer for 4 to 5 minutes then spread the hash evenly along the bottom of the pan and cook for 5 minutes until browned.

6. Scoop out four holes in the corned beef mixture then crack an egg into each hole.

7. Cook the eggs to the desired level then serve the corned beef hash with the eggs.

Apple Cinnamon Muffins

Servings: 10

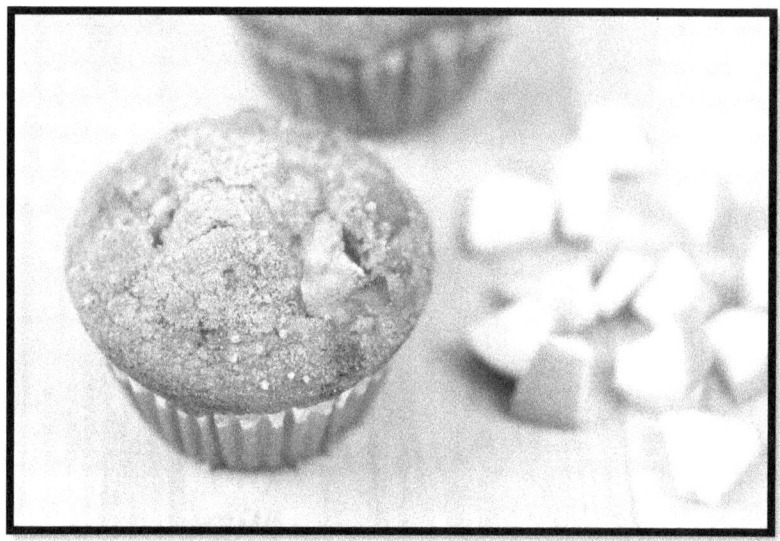

Ingredients:

- 1 cup almond flour
- ¼ cup coconut flour
- 1 tablespoon ground cinnamon
- ½ teaspoon baking soda
- 1/8 teaspoon salt
- 4 medium eggs, whisked
- ¼ cup coconut oil, melted
- 1 large green apple, cored and diced

Instructions:

1. Preheat the oven to 350°F and line a muffin pan with paper liners.
2. Combine the almond flour, coconut flour, cinnamon, baking soda and salt in a mixing bowl.
3. In a separate bowl, whisk together the eggs and coconut oil until smooth.
4. Add the wet ingredients to the dry and stir until smooth and well combined then fold in the apples.
5. Spoon the batter into the prepared pan, filling the cups about 2/3 full.
6. Bake for 25 to 30 minutes until a knife inserted in the center comes out clean.

7. Cool the muffins in the pan for 5 minutes then turn out onto a wire rack to cool completely.

Feta and Cherry Tomato Omelet

Servings: 1

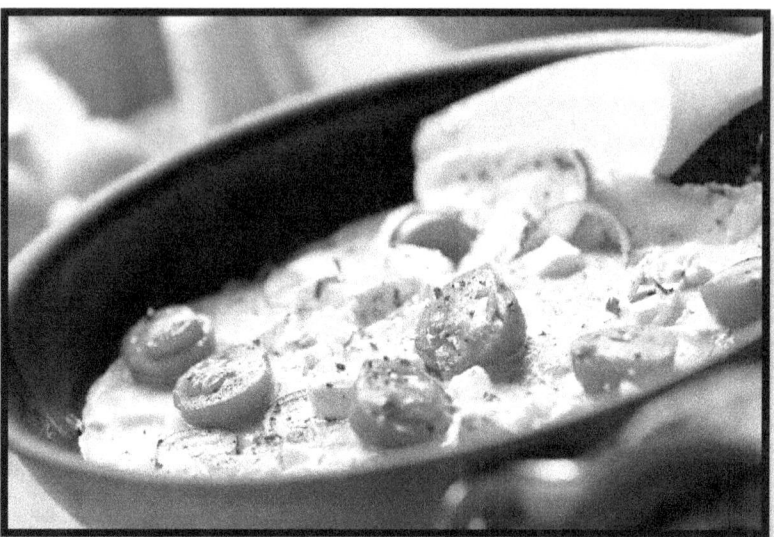

Ingredients:

- 2 large eggs
- 1 tablespoon whole milk
- Salt and pepper to taste
- 2 teaspoons olive oil
- ½ cup cherry tomatoes, halved
- 2 to 3 tablespoons crumbled feta cheese
- 1 thin slice red onion

Instructions:

1. Whisk together the eggs, milk, salt and pepper in a small bowl.
2. Heat 1 teaspoon oil in a small skillet over medium heat.
3. Add the tomatoes and cook for 2 minutes until tender.
4. Spoon the tomatoes into a bowl and set aside.
5. Add the remaining oil to the skillet and heat over medium-high heat.
6. Pour in the egg mixture and cook for 1 to 2 minutes until the egg begins to set.
7. Spoon the tomatoes over half the omelet and sprinkle the feta cheese on top.
8. Fold the empty half of the omelet over the filings and cook for 1 minute more until the egg is set.
9. Slide the omelet onto a plate and top with the sliced red onion to serve.

Carrot Green Apple Smoothie

Servings: 1 to 2

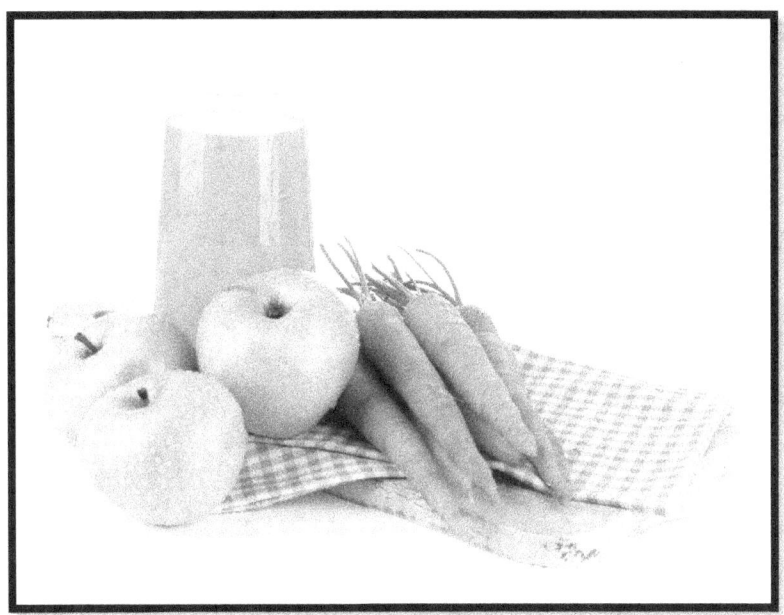

Ingredients:

- 2 small green apples, cored and chopped
- 1 medium carrot, peeled and chopped
- 1 cup water
- ½ cup ice cubes
- ¼ cup plain Greek yogurt
- Pinch ground ginger or cinnamon

Instructions:

1. Combine all of the ingredients in a blender.
2. Blend on high speed for 40 to 60 seconds until smooth.
3. Pour into a glass and serve immediately.

Classic Hummus

Servings: 6

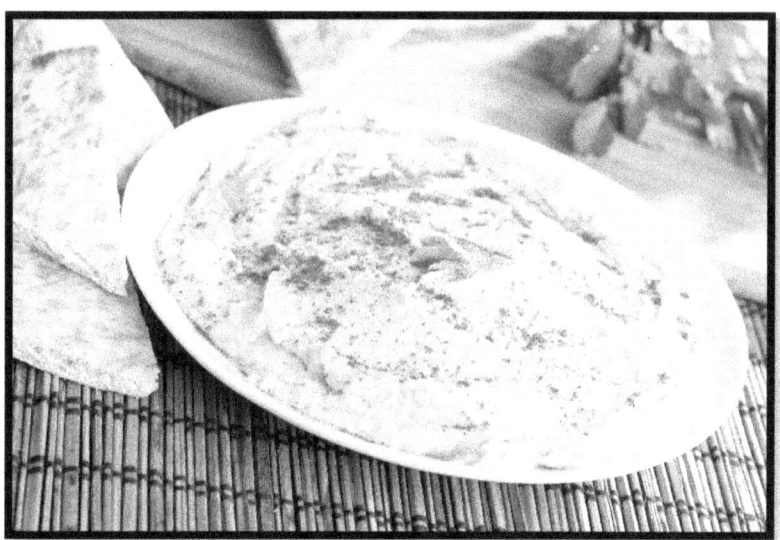

Ingredients:

- ¼ cup tahini
- Juice from 1 large lemon
- ½ teaspoon salt
- 2 tablespoons extra-virgin olive oil
- 1 small clove garlic, minced
- ¼ teaspoon ground cumin
- 1 (15 ounce) can chickpeas, rinsed and drained
- Water, as needed
- Pinch paprika

Instructions:

1. Combine the tahini, lemon juice and salt in a food processor.
2. Blend on high speed until smooth, about 60 seconds.
3. Add the olive oil, garlic, and cumin then blend for 30 seconds.
4. Scrape down the sides of the bowl and add the rinsed chickpeas.
5. Blend the mixture until smooth and creamy – add up to 3 tablespoons of water, if needed, to adjust the consistency.
6. Spoon the hummus into a bowl and sprinkle with paprika to serve.

Cream of Asparagus Soup

Servings: 4

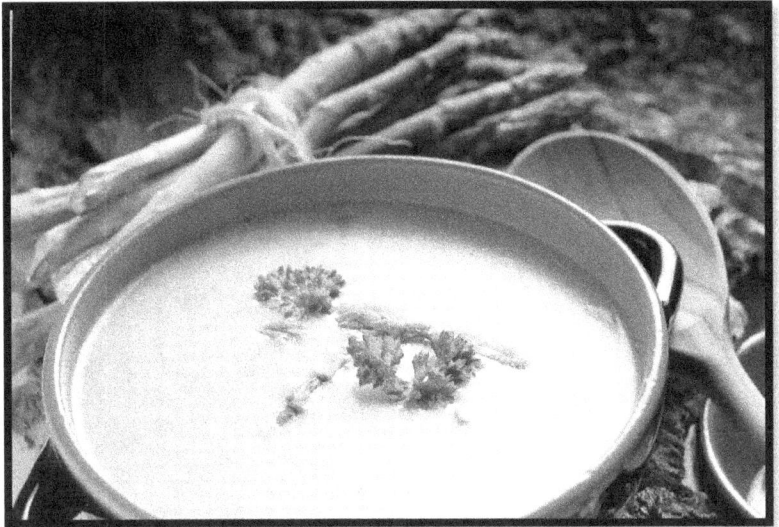

Ingredients:

- 1 tablespoon coconut oil
- 1 large leek, chopped (white and light green parts only)
- 4 cups chicken broth
- 1 large bunch asparagus, trimmed and cut into 1-inch chunks
- ¼ cup sour cream
- Salt and pepper to taste
- Fresh chopped parsley

Instructions:

1. Heat the oil in a stockpot over medium heat.
2. Add the leeks and cook for 8 to 10 minutes until tender.
3. Stir in the chicken broth and bring to a boil.
4. Reduce the heat to medium-low and stir in the asparagus – simmer for 12 to 15 minutes until tender.
5. Remove from heat then puree the soup using an immersion blender until smooth.
6. Return the pot to the heat and whisk in the sour cream, salt and pepper.
7. Serve hot, garnished with fresh chopped parsley.

Pesto Turkey Burgers

Servings: 4

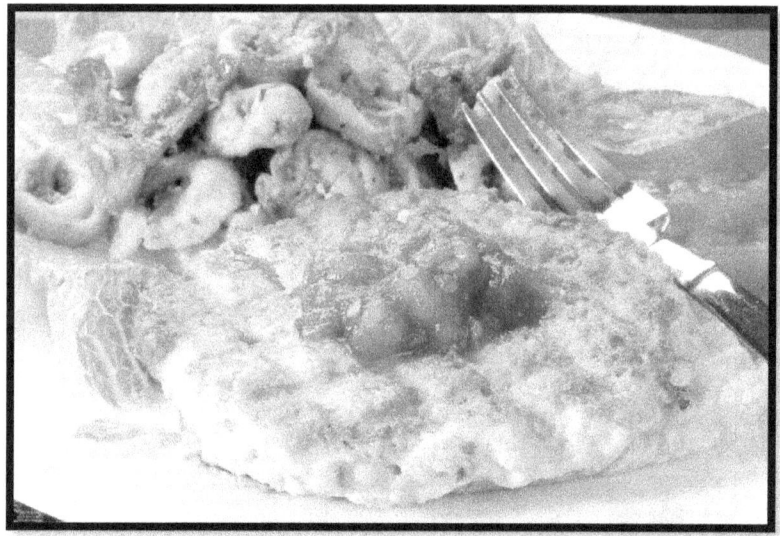

Ingredients:

- 1 ¼ lbs. lean ground turkey
- 1/3 cup homemade basil pesto
- Salt and pepper to taste

Instructions:

1. Preheat the broiler in your oven to high heat.
2. Combine the ground turkey and pesto in a mixing bowl along with the salt and pepper.
3. Shape the mixture into four even-sized patties, patting them to about ¾ inches thick.
4. Place the burgers on a broiler pan and cook for 4 to 5 minutes on each side until cooked through.
5. Serve the burgers hot on a bed of lettuce topped with your favorite burger toppings.

Cheesy Stuffed Mushrooms

Servings: 6 to 8

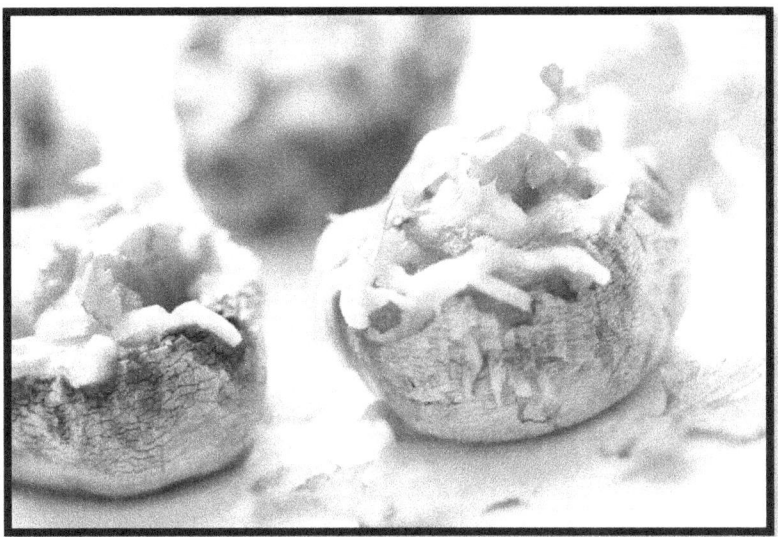

Ingredients:

- 1 ½ lbs. whole crimini mushrooms
- 2 tablespoons coconut oil
- ½ cup grated parmesan cheese
- 2 ounces cream cheese, softened
- Pinch ground pepper
- ¼ cup almond flour
- 1 teaspoon fresh chopped parsley

Instructions:

1. Preheat the oven to 350°F and line a rimmed baking sheet with parchment.
2. Remove the stems from the mushrooms and scrape the gills from each cap.
3. Clean the mushrooms with a damp paper towel then arrange upside down in the prepared baking sheet.
4. Chop the mushroom stems and combine with the onions in a mixing bowl.
5. Heat the oil in a skillet over medium heat.
6. Add the onion mixture and cook for 4 to 5 minutes until tender.
7. Turn off the heat then stir in the parmesan, cream cheese and black pepper.
8. Add ¼ cup almond flour and the parsley then spoon the mixture into the mushroom caps.
9. Bake for 25 minutes or until heated through. Serve hot.

Mixed Vegetable Curry

Servings: 6

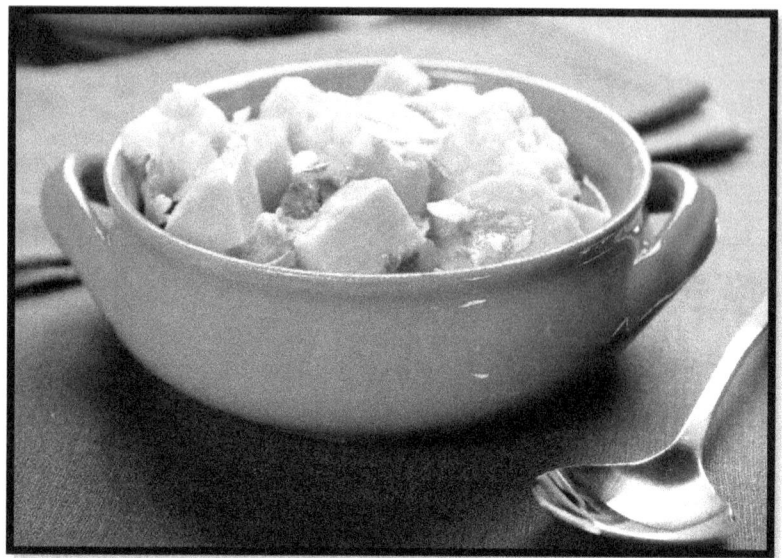

Ingredients:

- 2 tablespoons olive oil
- 1 tablespoon minced garlic
- 1 inch fresh ginger, grated
- 2 tablespoons curry powder
- 4 medium carrots, chopped
- 1 medium yellow onion, chopped
- 2 tablespoons tomato paste
- 1 (14.5 ounce) can diced tomatoes
- 2 cups chopped cauliflower florets
- 1 cup chopped broccoli florets
- 1 (14 ounce) can coconut milk
- Salt and pepper to taste
- ¼ cup fresh chopped cilantro

Instructions:

1. Heat the oil in a deep skillet over medium heat.
2. Add the garlic and ginger and cook for 2 minutes until fragrant.
3. Stir in the curry powder and cook for 1 minute more.

4. Add the carrots and onion and sauté for 6 to 8 minutes until the onions are translucent.
5. Stir in the tomato paste, tomatoes, broccoli, and cauliflower.
6. Simmer over medium heat for 12 to 15 minutes until the vegetables are tender.
7. Reduce heat to low and stir in the coconut milk.
8. Cook for 5 minutes or so over low heat until thickened.
9. Season with salt and pepper to taste.
10. Top with fresh chopped cilantro to serve.

Broiled Scallops with Orange Glaze

Servings: 4

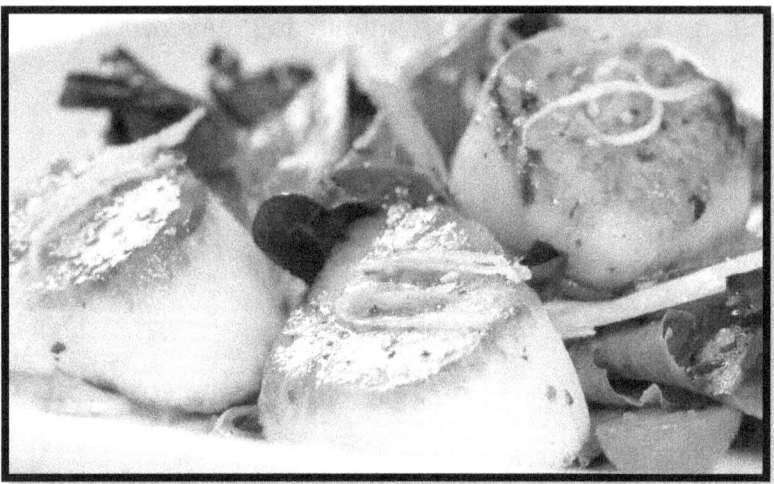

Ingredients:

- 1 lbs. raw sea scallops
- ¼ cup unsalted butter
- ½ cup fresh-squeezed orange juice
- 1 teaspoon minced garlic
- ¾ teaspoon salt
- ½ teaspoon pepper

Instructions:

1. Preheat the broiler in your oven to high heat.
2. Rinse the scallops in cool water then pat dry with paper towel.
3. Season the scallops with salt and pepper to taste.
4. Arrange the scallops on a broiler pan and broil for 2 to 3 minutes on each side until just cooked through.
5. Meanwhile, heat the butter in a small saucepan over medium-high heat.
6. Stir in the orange juice, garlic, salt and pepper.
7. Bring to a boil then reduce heat and simmer for 10 minutes.
8. Set aside to thicken while the scallops cook then drizzle over them to serve.

Chicken Brown Rice Soup

Servings: 6 to 8

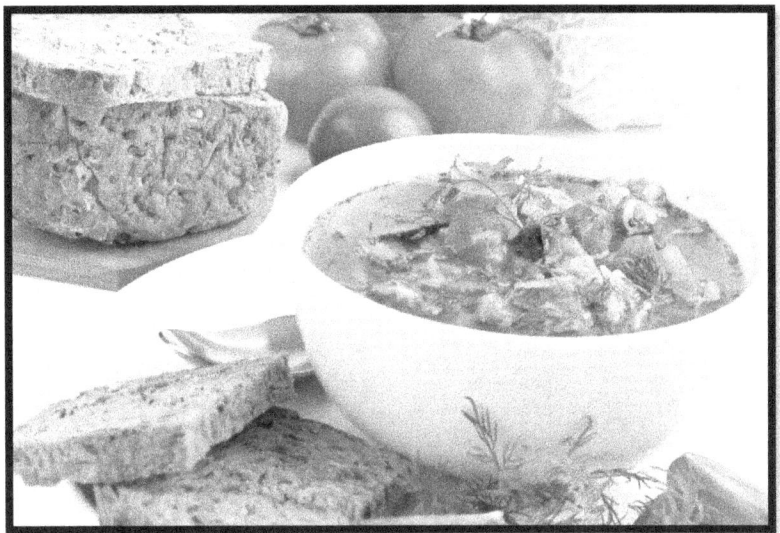

Ingredients:

- 8 cups chicken broth, divided
- 1 ½ cups diced carrot
- 1 large yellow onion, chopped
- 1 cup diced celery
- 2 cups water
- 1 boneless skinless chicken breast, chopped
- 1 cup brown rice, uncooked
- 1 bay leaf
- 3 cups fresh baby spinach
- Salt and pepper to taste

Instructions:

1. Bring ½ cup of broth to simmer in a stockpot.
2. Add the carrots, onion, and celery then simmer for 7 to 8 minutes until the onions are translucent.
3. Stir in the rest of the broth along with the water, chicken and rice.
4. Add the bay leaf then bring to a boil.
5. Reduce the heat and simmer, covered, for 30 to 35 minutes until the rice is tender.

6. Discard the bay leaf and stir in the spinach. Season with salt and pepper to taste.
7. Cook for 2 minutes until the spinach is wilted then serve hot.

Spinach Artichoke Dip

Servings: 6 to 8

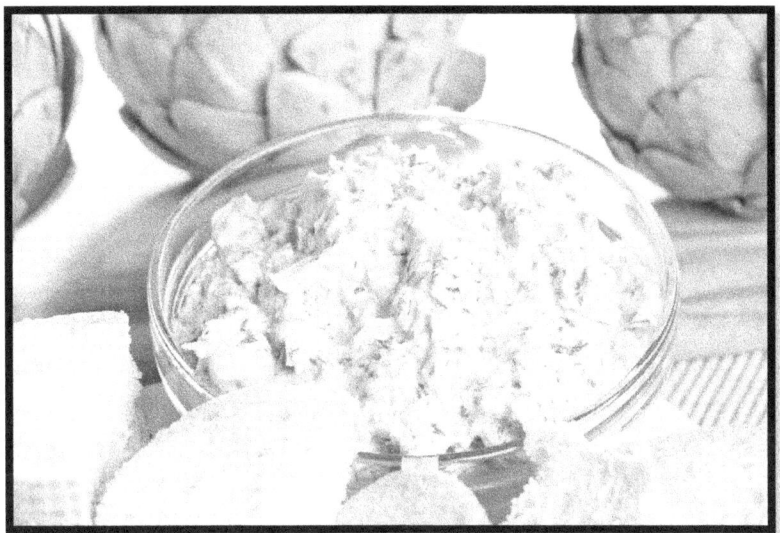

Ingredients:

- 2 cups shredded mozzarella cheese
- ½ cup sour cream
- 1 tablespoon minced garlic
- 1 (14 ounce) can artichoke hearts, drained and chopped
- 2 (8 ounce) blocks cream cheese, softened
- ½ (10 ounce) package frozen spinach, thawed and drained
- 3 tablespoons grated parmesan cheese

Instructions:

1. Preheat the oven to 350°F.
2. Stir together 1 ½ cups shredded mozzarella with the sour cream, garlic, artichoke hearts, cream cheese, and spinach in a mixing bowl.
3. Blend until well combined then spoon into a baking dish and sprinkle with parmesan and the remaining ½ cup mozzarella.
4. Bake for 30 minutes until hot and bubbling and browned on top.

Vegetarian Black Bean Burgers

Servings: 6

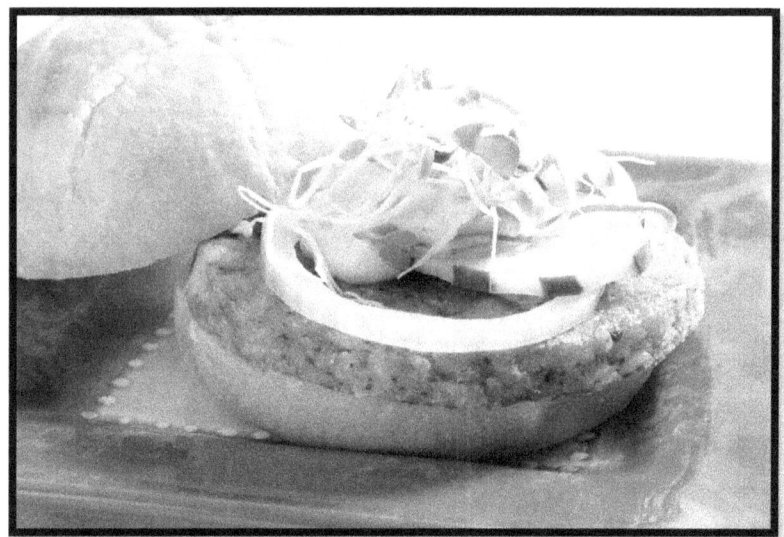

Ingredients:

- 1 (15 ounce) can black beans, rinsed and drained
- 1 large egg, whisked
- ½ small yellow onion, diced
- 1 cup almond flour
- ½ teaspoon garlic powder
- ½ teaspoon salt
- ¼ teaspoon black pepper
- 1 tablespoon olive oil

Instructions:

1. Pour the beans into a mixing bowl and mash gently with a fork or potato masher.
2. Stir in the egg, onion, almond flour, garlic powder, salt and pepper.
3. Blend the mixture until well combined then shape into 6 even-sized patties.
4. Heat the oil in a large skillet over medium-high heat.
5. Add the patties to the skillet and cook for 5 minutes on each side until heated through.
6. Serve hot on gluten-free buns topped with your favorite burger toppings.

Balsamic Grilled Salmon

Servings: 4

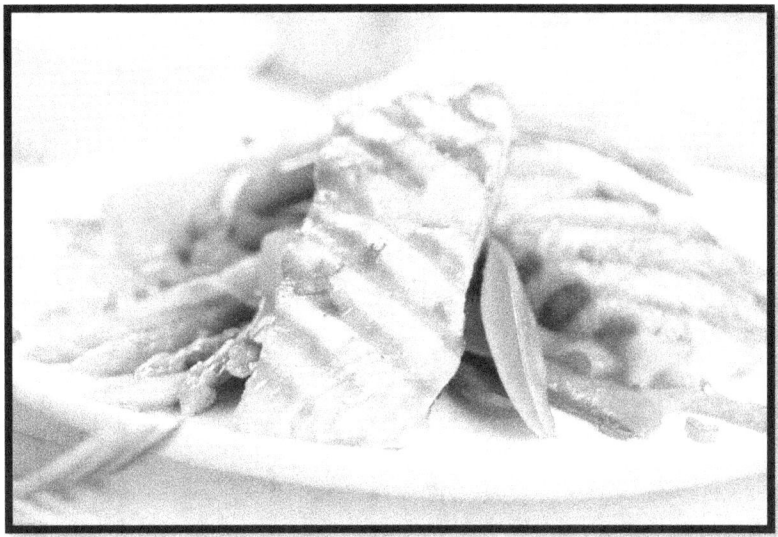

Ingredients:

- 4 (6 ounce) boneless salmon fillets
- 1/3 cup balsamic vinegar
- 1/3 cup dry white wine
- 1 ½ tablespoons fresh lemon juice
- Salt and pepper to taste

Instructions:

1. Preheat the grill to medium-high heat and brush the grates with olive oil.
2. Whisk together the balsamic vinegar, white wine and lemon juice in a small saucepan over medium heat.
3. Boil the mixture until it has reduced to about ¼ to 1/3 cup, about 15 minutes.
4. Season the fillets with salt and pepper to taste.
5. Place the fillets on the hot grill and cook for 4 to 5 minutes per side until just opaque in the center.
6. Transfer the salmon to a serving dish and drizzle with the balsamic glaze to serve.

Chilled Cucumber Mint Soup

Servings: 4

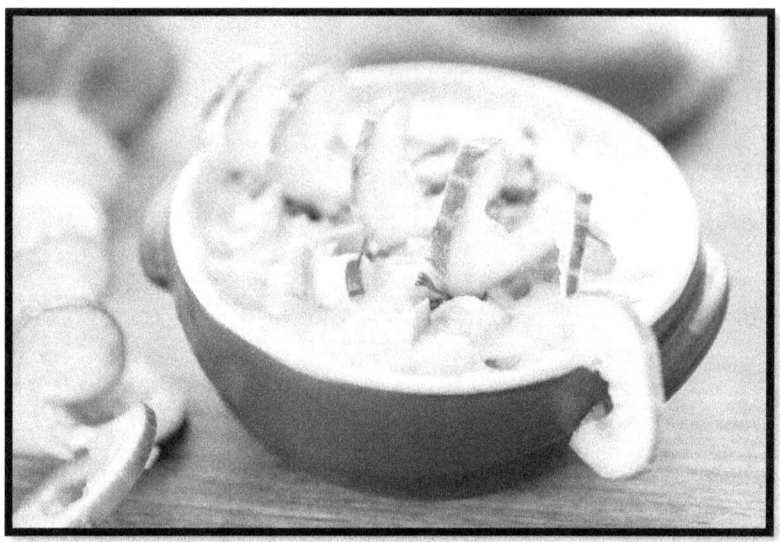

Ingredients:

- 1 ½ cups plain Greek yogurt
- ½ cup sour cream
- ¼ cup fresh chopped mint leaves
- 3 tablespoons fresh chopped parsley
- ½ cup sliced green onion
- 1 clove minced garlic
- Pinch salt and white ground pepper

Instructions:

1. Combine all of the ingredients in a food processor and blend smooth.
2. Pour the soup into a bowl then cover and chill for at least 3 hours.
3. Spoon into bowls and garnish with thinly sliced cucumber and fresh mint leaves to serve.

Basil Walnut Pesto

Servings: 8 to 10

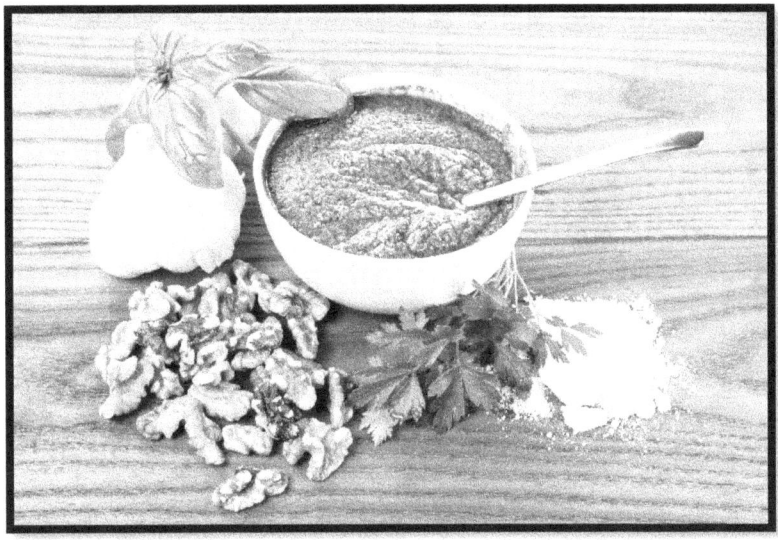

Ingredients:

- 2 cups fresh basil leaves, packed
- 2 ounces grated parmesan cheese
- 1/3 cup chopped walnuts
- 1 tablespoon minced garlic
- ½ cup extra-virgin olive oil
- Salt and pepper to taste

Instructions:

1. Combine the basil and walnuts in a food processor.
2. Pulse several times to chop then add the garlic and parmesan cheese.
3. Blend until smooth and combined then scrape down the sides of the bowl.
4. With the processor running, drizzle in the olive oil until the mixture is smooth.
5. Season with salt and pepper to taste.

Oven-Baked Haddock with Tomatoes

Servings: 4

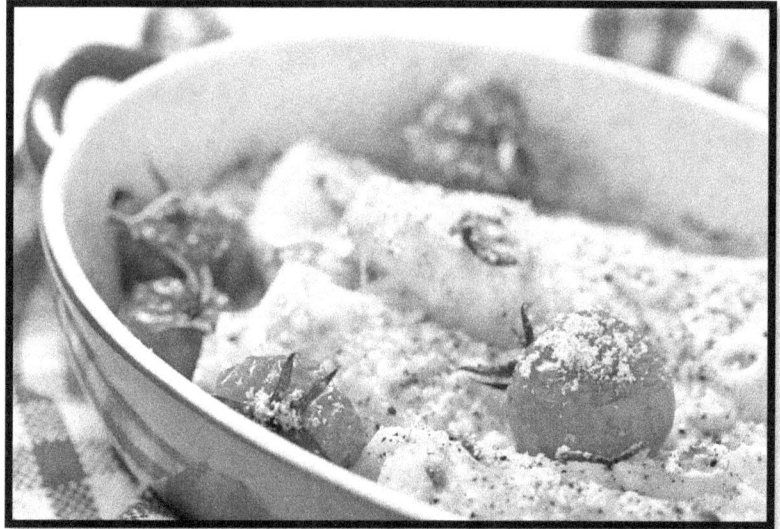

Ingredients:

- 4 (4 to 5 ounce) boneless haddock fillets
- Salt and pepper to taste
- 1 (15 ounce) can diced tomatoes, drained
- 3 tablespoons almond flour
- 1 teaspoon dried parsley

Instructions:

1. Preheat the oven to 350°F and lightly grease a casserole dish.
2. Rinse the fillets with cool water the pat dry.
3. Arrange the fillets in the casserole dish and season with salt and pepper to taste.
4. Pour the tomatoes into the dish around the fillets then sprinkle the almond flour and parsley over top of everything.
5. Bake for 18 to 25 minutes until the fillets are cooked through.

Baked Cabbage Rolls

Servings: 4

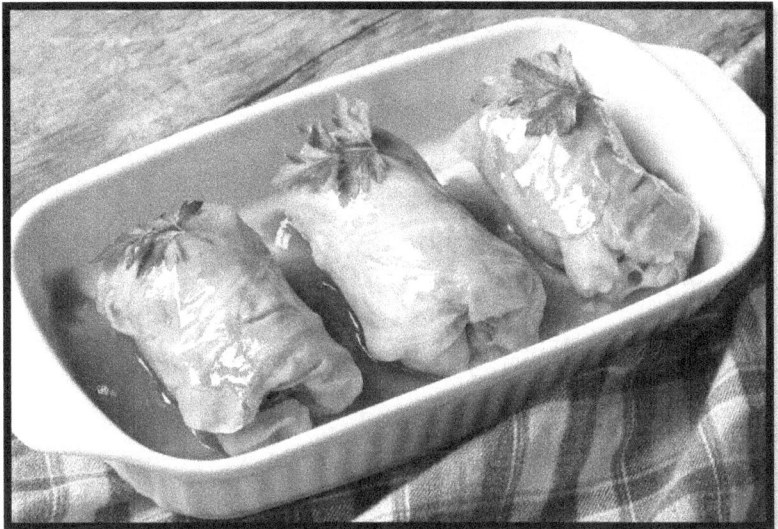

Ingredients:

- ½ large head cabbage, cored
- 2 teaspoons olive oil
- 1 large onion, diced
- 1 tablespoon minced garlic
- 2 cups canned crushed tomatoes
- 1 tablespoon apple cider vinegar
- ¾ cups cooked brown rice
- ½ lbs. lean ground beef
- 1 large egg
- Salt and pepper to taste

Instructions:

1. Bring a large pot of salted water to boil.
2. Add the cabbage, turning it often, until tender – about 15 to 18 minutes.
3. Remove the cabbage to a cutting board to drain then separate the leaves.
4. Select 10 of the largest leaves and trim away the ribs.
5. Preheat the oven to 375°F.
6. Heat the oil in a saucepot over medium-high heat.
7. Add the onions and cook for 4 to 5 minutes until tender.

8. Stir in the garlic and cook for 1 minute more.
9. Spoon half of the onion mixture into a mixing bowl then stir the tomatoes and vinegar into the saucepot.
10. Season with salt and pepper to taste then bring to a boil.
11. Reduce heat and simmer for 10 minutes.
12. Spread about 1 cup of the tomato sauce into a square baking dish.
13. Add the rice, ground beef, and egg to the onion mixture in the bowl.
14. Stir well and season with salt and pepper to taste.
15. Spoon some of the rice mixture into each of the reserved cabbage leaves, rolling the leaves around the filling.
16. Arrange the stuffed leaves in the baking dish and drizzle with the remaining tomato sauce.
17. Cover with foil then bake for 35 to 40 minutes.
18. Remove the foil then bake for another 10 minutes or until the sauce is bubbling.

Cinnamon Baked Apples

Servings: 2

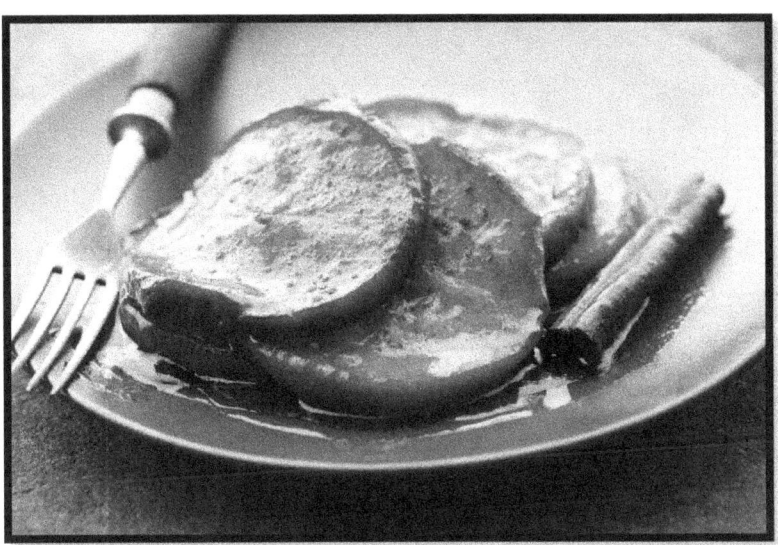

Ingredients:

- 2 large green apples, cored
- 2 tablespoons coconut oil
- 2 teaspoons ground cinnamon

Instructions:

1. Preheat the oven to 400°F.
2. Slice the apples to about 1/8 to ¼ inch thick.
3. Spread two pieces of foil onto a large baking sheet and arrange the apple slices on the foil.
4. Dot with pats of butter and sprinkle with cinnamon.
5. Fold the foil up around the apple slices into two packets.
6. Bake for 25 minutes until the apples are tender.

Bittersweet Chocolate Mousse

Servings: 2

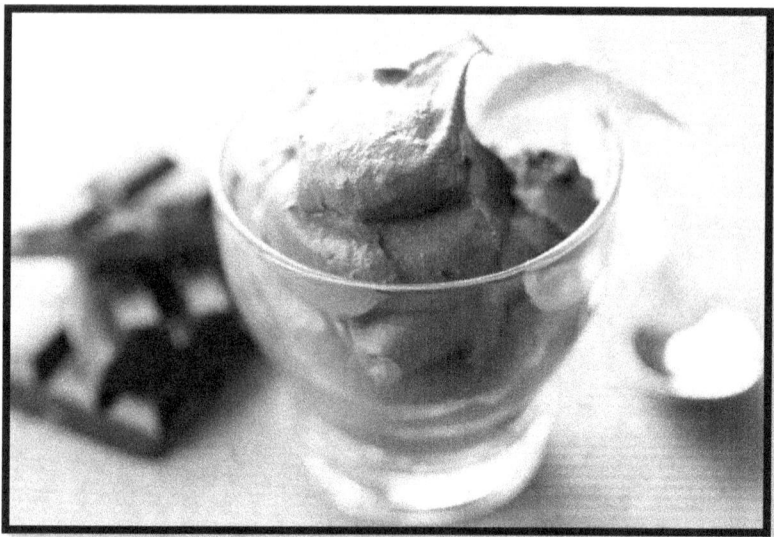

Ingredients:

- 1 large ripe avocado, pitted and chopped
- 2 tablespoons unsweetened cocoa powder
- ¼ teaspoon vanilla extract

Instructions:

1. Combine the ingredients in a food processor.
2. Blend until smooth and creamy then spoon into dessert bowls.
3. Chill until ready to serve, at least 1 hour.

Almond Apple Crisp

Servings: 6

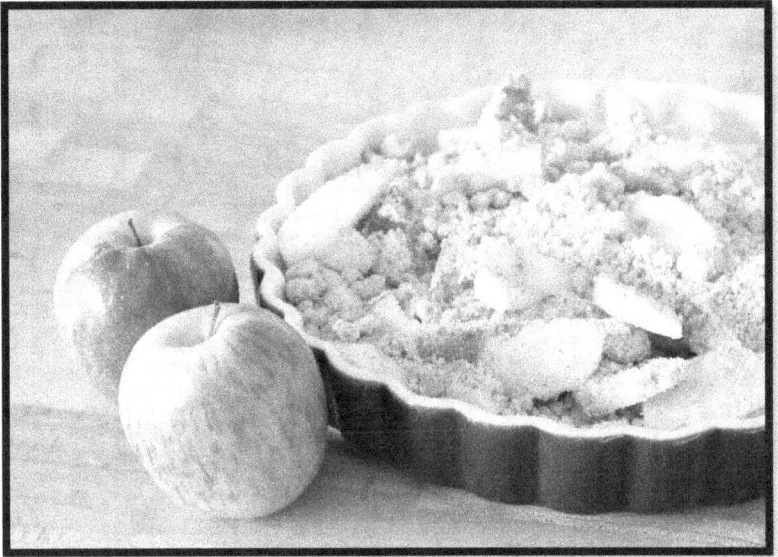

Ingredients:

- 3 large green apples, cored and sliced thin
- 2 tablespoons fresh lemon juice
- 1 ¼ cups almond flour
- ¼ cup finely chopped almonds
- ¼ cup shredded unsweetened coconut
- 1 ½ tablespoons ground cinnamon
- ¼ cup melted coconut oil

Instructions:

1. Preheat the oven to 300°F.
2. Spread the apples in the bottom of a square glass baking dish.
3. Drizzle with lemon juice.
4. Combine the almond flour, almonds, coconut, and cinnamon in a mixing bowl.
5. Add the melted coconut oil and stir until it forms a crumbled mixture.
6. Sprinkle the mixture over the apples and cook for 45 minutes until hot and bubbling.
7. Let the apple crisp cool for 10 minutes before serving.

Conclusion

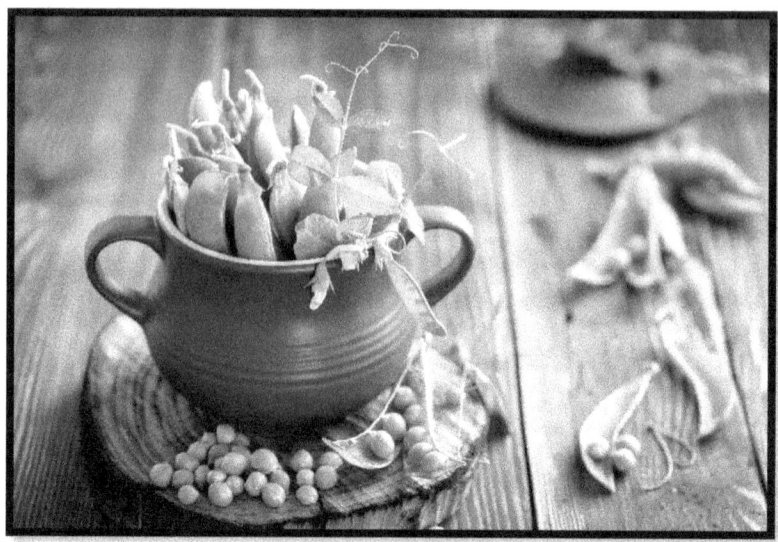

After reading this book, you should know and understand the basics of what a sugar detox diet is and how it can benefit you. While giving up sugar may seem like a daunting task, the recipes in this book are proof that it doesn't have to be torturous. In fact, you may find it easier than you think! In no time at all, you will start to feel the benefits of removing sugar from your diet and you will not look back. So, take the information you learned from this book, along with the tasty recipes, and get started – you won't regret it!